The Promise
PREMATURELY DELAYED

A Couple's Journey of Hope for Starting a Family

The Promise
PREMATURELY DELAYED

A Couple's Journey
of Hope for
Starting a Family

Joseph & Pamela Bowman

Hunter Heart Publishing
Colorado Springs, Colorado

The Promise: Prematurely Delayed
Copyright © October 2015
by Joseph and Pamela Bowman

First Edition

All rights reserved. No part of this book may be reproduced or transmitted in any form or by any means without written permission of the author or publisher. Scripture is taken from the New American Standard Bible (NASB) Copyright © 1960, 1962, 1963, 1968, 1971, 1972, 1973, 1975, 1977, 1995 by The Lockman Foundation .

To order products, bulk issue, or for any other correspondence:

Hunter Heart Publishing
4164 Austin Bluffs Parkway, Suite 214
Colorado Springs, Colorado 80918
www.hunterheartpublishing.com
Tel. (253) 906-2160 – Fax: (719) 368-6655
E-mail: publisher@hunterheartpublishing.com
Or reach us on the internet: www.hunterheartpublishing.com
"Offering God's Heart to a Dying World"

This book and all other Hunter Heart Publishing™ Eagle's Wings Press™ and Hunter Heart Kids™ books are available at Christian bookstores and distributors worldwide.

Chief Editor: Gord Dormer
Book cover design:
Phil Coles Independent Design
Layout & logos: Exousia Marketing Group www.exousiamg.com
ISBN: 978-1-937741-61-7
Printed in the United States of America

This Book Is Dedicated:

To our 4 miracles,

Joseph – Josiah – Jewell – Joshua

and…

To all couples who are hoping, praying and waiting for little "promises"!

Acknowledgments

Our Parents, in alphabetical order: Joseph S. Bowman III, Melba Jean Harrison, Reginal & Lisa Macklin and Alfred & Linda Roberson

Our Grandparents, Edna E. Travis, Johnny & Dorothy Sims, John Owens, Jewell Fawlkes Bowman, Joseph S. Bowman II, Elvin Roberson, Melvin Harrison, Charlene Trotter-Harrison (Light Gray Deceased)

Dr. Mildred Spencer, Dr. A.P. Barker , Drs. William & Marj Wolfson, Dr. James McHugh, Dr. Richard Agress, Dr. Reginald Kendall, Dr. Josephine H. Amory, Swedish Medical Center, Daisha Scarlett, Kimberly Dunn, "Mama" Kim Thurman, Curtis Wade, B. Dwayne Hardin, Beverly Hubbard, Mr. Cecil McKenzie

John & Karina Blasco, Willie & Tajuana Davidson, Phillip & Taisha Moore Lester & LaTrisha Kinlow, Eugene & Wanda Garrett, Michael & Tanisha Roberts, Benjamin Singleton and the entire Integrity Life Church Family, Nia Grant, Leah Shephard, Myrtice Walker, Mother Alice Avery, Uncle Willie Mills, Lady Laura Witherspoon, Mostly Muffins Inc., Financial Pacific Leasing LLC, Federal Way Public Schools

Mssy. Debbie Jones, Mssy. Gwendolyn Townsend, Maketa Brazier, Kim "Nana" Moore, Renolda "CoCo" Grant, Pastor

Jerry Jones, Dr. Dermathe LaVelle, Charleen Lacy, and our entire family and loving friends.

"The Village" of Babysitters for the Bowman Children: Auntie Portia Roberson, Vikki Polk, Toya Williams, Heather Fountain, Courtney Jenkins, Telisha Perryman, Christina Wiley, Mom Joyce Womack, Carolyn Blanchey

In Memoriam

Talethia Bible
William Watson
Pastor William Smith
Myles Corrigan
Mother Hazel White
Ajiah Matthews
Mother Stella Scott
Rosemary Blasco

Foreword

The first time I met Joseph and Pamela Bowman, I immediately knew there was something special about this extraordinary couple and their powerful faith. Pamela shared her story with me about the many years of trying to have a child. When J-5 was born at 24 weeks weighing under two pounds, Pamela said to me, "We believe this is a blessing. This child is a miracle." Her strength and faith in God were unwavering and she had this magical way of finding the good in this traumatic and extremely emotional situation. She told me, "We are thankful to get this far."

Pamela's words have stayed with me. Their story will inspire me for life. I have been a Parent Mentor for families with babies in the NICU for ten years, and I have shared Pamela and Joseph's story to inspire many distraught and frightened parents. I also had an extremely premature son born at 26 weeks gestation in 1994. I understand how difficult having a child in the NICU can be and my goal as a mentor is to bring comfort and hope to parents during this time. God blessed me with the opportunity to share J-5's journey with this prayerful, positive, and loving couple.

Pamela came to the NICU every day dressed in nice outfits and matching jewelry. She would sit next to J-5's isolette and say prayers, or sing a soft song. She was a beautiful mother, proud to be with her son. She would greet everyone with a warm smile and you could just feel the grace of God being passed onto you. In this book, Pamela and Joseph will inspire, give hope, and pass on a story that makes you never want to give up on your dreams.

Annette Alling
March of Dimes Parent Mentor and friend of Pamela and Joseph

Table of Contents

Chapter One: In The Beginning 1

Chapter Two: Where Are the Little Ones? 5

Chapter Three: The Sojourn 7

Chapter Four: One In The Oven 11

Chapter Five: The Royal Flush 13

Chapter Six: The Big "Sweed" 17

Chapter Seven: Finally Home 23

Chapter Eight: An Encore Performance 25

Chapter Nine: Playing With Fire 27

Chapter Ten: Never Give Up: Promise Keeper 31

About the Author 37
Scriptures 39
Bibliography 41

Chapter One

IN THE BEGINNING

In 1995, Pam and I reconnected at South Seattle Community College via a failed college football journey. I (Joseph) migrated from Pacific Lutheran University and enrolled at the community college where my father was an instructor. Pam had all intents to travel "down south" for college; nonetheless, she was renewing her life after a failed marriage of one year and landed at the same educational institution. One day, while I was walking the campus to register for classes, I saw Pam in the distance and greeted her with the following: "How are your parents? How is the married life?" She quickly responded with "They're doing great!" and "That's over." We began to converse and catch up on "old times," remembering as far back as our grandmothers worshipping together in the same church in the 60's. Our parents subsequently led churches in their generation, as well. Catching up involved "remember when's" and the proverbial "ideal life" dialogue. We convened under the campus' tower clock as Joe and Pam, the young kids from church, leaving with the realization that we were both migrating from the paralyzing jaws of disappointment.

From that day forward, we continued to strengthen our connection. In December of 1995, we had a euphoric moment surrounded by the chill from Lake Washington and the bliss of Christmas was in the air. We embraced under the stars, and in that moment, it felt as if Heaven and all its angels stopped and applauded this moment of love.

On June 28, 1997, we married and set our lives on a journey of greatness in continuing the legacy so graciously modeled before us. Through three generations of our families being connected, who would have known that we would be blessed to fall in love and be united in holy matrimony with over five hundred witnesses! What a wonderful day that was! With the uniting of two local "well-knows," the expectation was for us to produce more generations to make more robust the pedigree of greatness. Consequently, our fruit seemed to be barren. I mean - no pressure or anything; we were the bonding agent for three generations of impactful, religious leaders. In addition, I am Joseph S. Bowman IV (4th) which means the "V" (5th) was MANDATORY!

Our first "life" project as a couple was investing into 375 kids over a period of twelve years through the vehicle of music & academic empowerment. The group (Youth For Christ Shebach Choir) sang for diplomats, juvenile facilities, schools, and multi-platinum recording artists. In addition, we recorded two CD's of our own. We invested our lives into the youth weekly; the outpost was a singing group, however, in reality, we created an environment to incubate great leaders of tomorrow. We will be forever grateful to Melba Jean Harrison (Pam's Mom) for her investment in envisioning an opportunity for us to grow, as well as the kids.

We gathered to sing, but the truth was we were teaching them life skills, while investing into them in a great way and awakening their understanding to the fruitfulness of life. Some of the academic empowerment events that we engaged were annual retreats, summer tours, singing for corporate events and recording at Seattle's fine Benoroya Hall.

We both worked full-time jobs; Joseph continued his education and hosted a weekly gospel radio show on Sundays. He also served as a deacon in the church, while I continued writing music and singing at special events in the community and abroad, I was also the director of our church choir. Nonetheless, with all the busyness surrounding us, we were very focused on having our own children.

What we hold fast to be true is dedicated service and going the extra mile, pouring out yourself and giving all you have for someone else, submitting yourself to the dispossessed and those who are in despair, ministering to the down and out and down and up is truly the opportunity of a lifetime. What rests in that opportunity is grace and favor on your life and greater opportunity will come to you. The great investment will pay off.

So this is our journey through triumph, struggle, faith and honor. Please open your heart to journey with us—a story that never gets old—not to us, at least. By no means is our story the only one of its type; however, our goal is to raise hope and to catapult you to a greater YOU!

Chapter Two

WHERE ARE THE LITTLE ONES?

Everywhere we went the question would always arise from family and friends, "Where are the little ones?" This was a devastating question after so many years. Year one was okay, year two, maybe, year six and seven, but by year eight and nine, it became very arduous in the process of life for us and reflected some real disheartening probabilities.

As a little girl, I recall playing with my dolls and acting as if I was a wife and mommy. I would get lost in combing my doll's hair, dressing her, cooking in my easy-bake oven and actually preparing for motherhood. I can clearly see myself looking out of the window in my bedroom at this big, pretty tree that seemed to touch the sky. That tree was a direct connection to Heaven in my childlike mind. I would look up into the clouds and say this prayer often, "Dear God, it's me Pam and I thank you for blessing me with a nice, loving, handsome, hardworking husband and beautiful babies one day…Oh and a nice big house in Jesus Name, Amen." Time went on and I was so elated that God had blessed me with two of my requests, but hadn't touched the other. After having years of blissful marriage resulting in no children became beyond devastating.

With Joseph and I being very active in our communities and coming from families well known in our state and abroad, it became extremely difficult to face the constant questions, "When will you have children? Is there something wrong? Are you not doing it right? What's the issue???" We smiled through it all, as we had become accustomed to it.

There were many times that I would take pregnancy tests in hopes that we were pregnant, because all of the signs and symptoms were there. We should have been the smiling Africa American couple for pregnancy test commercials.

I constantly received baby shower invitations and would attend smiling through my tears, while congratulating the expectant mothers. It wasn't that I was not sincerely happy for them; I just couldn't put my finger on why it was taking me forever to get pregnant. I recall going to my car after leaving, sitting there balling in tears. My faith was great in every area, until it came to this. It became very difficult to fathom why we weren't pregnant, especially after pouring and investing into the lives of so many young people for so many years. I remember thinking to myself, surely if we had a cross to bear, this would not be it. I must admit my faith was almost non-existent and my heart was broken in pieces. I can't describe the torment that plagued me knowing that we hadn't conceived.

As time passed along we continued taking pregnancy tests. We would always say, "This time is going to be different." Yet and still, the tests came out negative. The pain on a scale from 0-10 was an 11, such a feeling of failure, disappointment and emptiness.

Chapter Three

THE SOJOURN

Pam and I are believers that great things come to fruition; consequently, we do understand it will not happen by osmosis. To that fact, we understood we needed to consult with some of the best physicians in the area. For the sake of their privacy, we will note them as Dr. L., Dr. M. and Dr. K. In year six, we sought medical advice from Pam's childhood and primary physician Dr. M. We discussed different options concerning our probability to conceive. After six years of using no form of contraception or birth control, we wanted answers. We were reasonably overcome by the unknown. So not only did we want answers, we blazed a trail to solving this mystery.

Upon taking Dr. M's advice, we consulted with a series of specialized physicians. Our first step on the journey was a consultation with Dr. K. a highly respected OBGYN who serviced many of our family members. He had a long dialogue with us concerning greater health decisions to include; losing weight, getting more sleep and the other negative components that can prohibit optimal health. The appointment seemed timeless as most of the conversation surrounded old family memories.

He gave us a prescription for life, one you can't fulfill at your local pharmacy. He stated, "Do your part to prepare, and the rest will happen on its own." We continued our journey with Dr. L., a renowned fertility specialist who proficiently examined and ordered ultrasound photos to reveal the facts. It was Valentine's Day 2005 that we arrived at our second visit to gain the results. We had extreme nerves in our stomach. We sat down and the information was incriminating against us to this fact; medical science had reached a conclusion concerning our situation. The following words shook the room, "Mrs. Bowman, it is nearly impossible that you will ever conceive a child."

In defense of this prolific medical doctor, the evidence was laid before us. He showed on the ultrasound pictures that Pam's ovaries were the size of a uterus and her uterus was the size of an ovary. He stated this is a result of a fertility drug given to women in the 70's called Diethylstilbestrol. From about 1940 to 1970, DES was given to pregnant women in the mistaken belief it would reduce the risk of pregnancy complications and losses. In 1971, DES was shown to cause a rare vaginal tumor in girls and women who had been exposed to this drug in utero.

The United States Food and Drug Administration subsequently withdrew DES from use in pregnant women. Follow-up studies have indicated DES also has the potential to cause a variety of significant adverse medical complications during the lifetime of girls who were exposed to it. After two years of carrying the weight of this diagnosis, we still continued to believe for a miracle. We went so far as to purchasing baby bottles, clothes and bibs, strategically placing them as if we were really parenting.

The Promise: Prematurely Delayed

It was Palm Sunday of 2007 and we once again surrendered ourselves to ANOTHER pregnancy test that often resulted negative. I was complaining about stomach cramping and pain for over two weeks. Joseph told me he was going to the gym and he'd return with a pregnancy test or give me a free limousine ride to the local hospital. I dreaded the "absolutely no" for the 20+ occurrence. I was filled with the dread of disappointment, however, I reached deep in my soul for the strength to endure the process, hopefully by now resulting in a "positive" YES! I rendered the bodily fluids necessary to formulate the test. I placed the test out of sight for about ten minutes. Too anxious for the jury to deliver a verdict, I asked Joseph to discover the results. He stated the "-" was decisive, however, the "positive" required "-" and "+". Again, the negative was clear and the positive was faint enough at least for us to pay attention. We placed it back in the bathroom pantry as the encasing plastic of the apparatus was explosive. We revisited the evidence to find the outcome of the test was POSITIVE!

We called our parents and a few choice friends around midnight to exclaim, "We think we're pregnant," super excited and extremely cautious. We made an appointment with my family doctor who took yet another urine sample. We waited with baited breath for the official results. The doctor walked around the corner and gave us two thumbs up. We cheered, hugged and cried. After ten years, the Bowman's were finally pregnant.

Chapter Four

One in the Oven

Upon confirming the little Bowman embryo was a living seed, we began sharing the news with the whole world. For our internal and external communities, it was as if the paparazzi released the information to the producers of "TMZ". The word spread via social media and word of mouth so fast, we received many calls congratulating us. I (Pam) made it through the first month just fine. Of course, keeping my appointments as directed, until one day, we found ourselves settling a domestic dispute (physical altercation) at church between a newlywed couple. Upon arriving home, I noticed "spotting," which usually indicates an issue with the pregnancy. I called early Monday morning to speak with my OBGYN, and he responsibly scheduled an appointment for me the same day to see what was going on. Upon his exam, I recall his verbal expression to be "Ahhhhhhhhh," as he exclaimed to me he could visibly see the membrane around Baby Joseph. He scheduled me for an immediate surgery (McDonald Cerclage) in a suspense position to ensure Baby Joseph would remain safe and secure for the remainder of the pregnancy. A McDonald Cerclage, described in 1957 is the most common, and is essentially a purse string stitch used to cinch the cervix shut; the cervix stitching involves a band of suture at the upper part of the cervix, while the lower part has already started to efface. This cerclage is usually placed between 12 weeks and 14 weeks of pregnancy. The stitch is generally removed around the 37th week of gestation. [5] This procedure was the literal hem stitch between life and death for the highly anticipated baby due November 15th.

With this only being June, I was surrendered to bed-rest with the exceptions of ultrasound appointments and bathroom breaks ONLY. At twenty-two weeks, my doctor commissioned me to the ante partum unit of the hospital for support just in case the baby required delivery. I sat there in the hospital "day-in" and "day-out" with Joseph by my side sleeping on a hospital cot, going to work each morning from my bed-side. One of the perinatal doctors said, "I'm going to give you a series of shots to help the baby's respiratory development." As he walked out of the room, he paused and turned and confidently said, "I think the baby will be born in about seven days." Joseph and I looked with disbelief as I was only 23 weeks along – a vast majority of medical facilities won't attempt to maintain a baby less than 24 weeks in utero. We began counting down the days of strict suspension to the orders of doctors and nurses for optimal care for Baby Joseph and me.

Chapter Five

The Royal Flush

Wednesday night, (July 25th) I kept feeling "something" as it pertained to the baby's movement and constantly told my nurse that something was happening. After checking the position of my cervix multiple times, it was determined that all was well and the cerclage was still in place. The day went on into the night and this sensation continued. Around 5:00 am, I felt a strong urge to use the restroom. I literally heard a loud voice say, "Get up and try to use the restroom before Joseph leaves for work." I had just got into a comfortable position and was reluctant to move, but I did. I got up and migrated to the restroom and while sitting there, I had this overwhelming feeling of unwarranted anticipation that I was in for the surprise of my life.

After several moments in building the courage to return to my bed, I stood to sanitize from urinating and in doing so, I felt an unidentified object below. I began to familiarize myself with what looked like the foot of the baby. Keep in mind, my visualization was limited due to my protruding stomach. I stood and looked in the mirror and what reflected back to me was Baby Joseph's entire foot dangling out of my birth canal. I waddled two steps out of the bathroom and yelled, "Big Joseph,

Little Joseph is trying to escape!" Joseph pulled the emergency string that on this occurrence, seemed to be stuck. He also attempted to dial the nurse from the television remote, while holding me and trying to avoid slipping on the embryonic fluid.

This moment of 120 seconds seemed like an eternity. I finally got Pam settled and grabbed the very responsible nurses and they went into full action; consistent to the nature of their care. Ironically, Baby Joseph's timing was impeccable, as I had briefcase in hand on my way to work. The nurses wheeled Pam to the operating room to prep for surgery. The skilled Dr. A. had to make a split-second decision to deliver Baby Joseph vaginally, instead of a Cesarean section, as he was extremely premature and breech.

I (Joseph) recall the nurses preparing me with scrubs and then instructing me to sit for a moment until they returned. In that moment, I asked God for His strength for Pam and Baby Joseph. As I sat there on a transport hospital bed up against the wall, such a peace surrounded me. It was literally that peace that guided my heart and mind (Phil 4:7). As I entered the room, I felt like there would be no defeat, because God was with Pam and I and most of all, with Baby Joseph. With a team of skilled doctors and nurses, Baby Joseph made his entrance into the world at a whopping 1lb. and 3oz. I kissed Pam, as she was to undergo surgery to repair her birth canal from the rigorous delivery. I (Joseph) went with Baby Joseph to the Neonatal Intensive Care Unit and another skilled team was anticipating his arrival. I saw my first born son (**The Promise**) laying there with arms flailing and legs kicking with oxygen being administered over his little face with a multitude of tubes, and being relegated to a "Rolls Royce" of an incubator. Joseph S. Bowman

V had arrived with a bruised left (the escape) leg, translucent skin, a head full of hair and an oversized diaper! I (Pam) still recall being medicated and told to look at our son quickly. All I remember is looking at him saying, "He's so strikingly handsome and little!" Maybe a second after that, Little Joseph put his thumb up as if to say, "Mommy, I'm going to be just fine." It was then that I knew and rested in the fact that God had everything in full control.

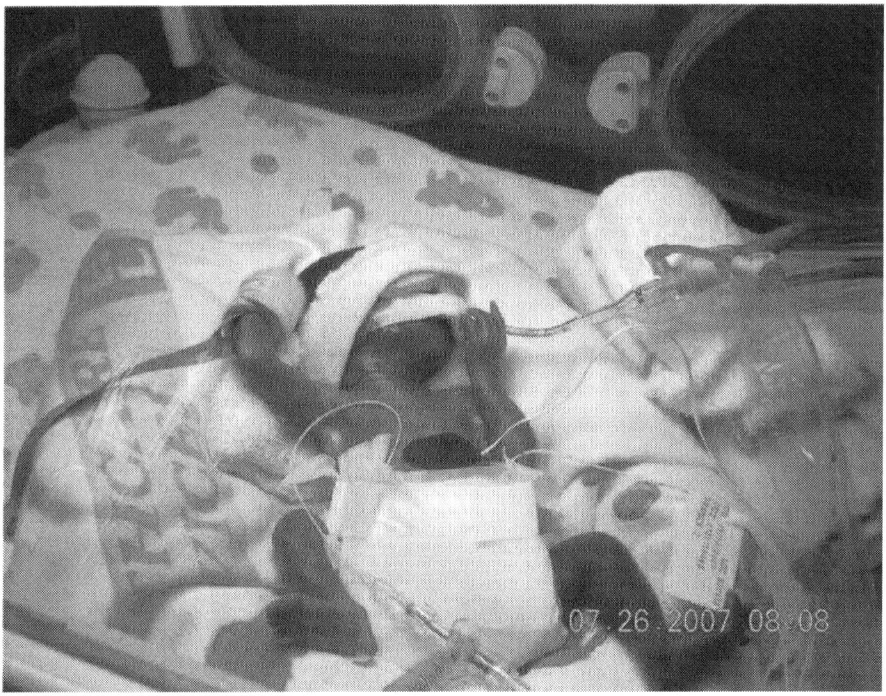
07.26.2007 08:08

Chapter Six

The Big "Sweed"

After the conclusion of my (Pam) surgery, I remember waking up in a brightly lit room thinking to myself; what in the world just happened! I was fully aware that I delivered Baby Joseph, but was still unsure as to the details. After seeing Joseph and receiving love and kudos from him, the next person I saw was my God Sister Tammy Atkins, who was one of the first people to see our little miracle. Seeing her was another sign that all was well, as she always brings a smile to my face and joy to my heart.

Because things happened so quickly, we were unable to notify our parents, family and friends of what had taken place. I remember hearing Joseph on the phone as he called our parents first and explained that the baby was just born. All I could hear was, "You've got to be kidding me….REALLY….are they okay?" Of course, it was just a matter of minutes before our parents arrived–two other family members had just flown out to the annual family reunion the day prior. Word traveled fast both near and far that Baby Bowman had arrived! We nearly had seventy-five visitors the first day! After getting myself (Pam) together, I took a ride via my chariot (wheel chair) entered the door of the NICU and saw my precious baby boy. There are no words that can describe the feeling that overcame me. It was as if he knew I was his mommy and I was there with him. Time stood still for a few moments and I began to thank God for his safe arrival and told him that I would be there with him every single day. This was a promise that I kept to him! I would have cherished the moment just to hold him in my arms; however, he was just too fragile to be handled. After being in the hospital four days, it was time for me to go home. I WAS NOT prepared to leave the hospital without my baby. It hit me like a ton of bricks, as I began to pack my bags in preparation to leave. I recall Joseph and I going up to tell little Joseph that we were leaving and would be back in the morning to see him. It was then that it really hit home. I was leaving the hospital and not taking my baby with me! As we drove away, tears began to fall like raindrops. I wanted to spend every waking moment there with my baby, but I knew that he was where he needed to be and would receive the best care. Needless to say, that was a LONG, restless night. The journey of getting up, getting ready and going to the hospital while Joseph went to work became our everyday routine. The hospital was twenty-two miles away from our home but there was no distance or time that could keep us from seeing our miracle. During this process, God sent us an angel in the form of our Uncle, Willie Mills, who so graciously drove me to the hospital several days, as Joseph was working. He shared words of inspiration, faith and joy as we traveled down Interstate-5. We will forever be grateful for his loving-kindness shown towards us.

The nurses and staff would often mention how shocked they were that I (Pam) was able to come there daily looking like a million bucks! It was important to me to present myself as victorious and triumphant, both inside and out. I realized that our son counted on me having a positive outlook and mindset not only for myself, but more so for him. I worked really hard to surrender my emotions for his success.

I knew baby Joseph's nourishment was essential while in the hospital and quickly found out that I would be fully responsible for pumping breast milk. He was being tube-fed on a daily basis. The act of pumping had to be done every day, three to four times a day. There was actually a "pump room" next to the NICU (Neonatal Intensive Care Unit) where I met other women that shared this awesome task. I must admit, I've never milked a cow, but I can sure imagine how she feels.

Baby Joseph was in the hospital 105 long days and no matter how I felt, I was there every single day! Joseph would come to the hospital after work, so that we could both spend time with the baby. This period of time was very intense, exciting and sometimes challenging. The nurses prepared us for what would be an emotional rollercoaster ride, but we didn't really know what was ahead for us, until we started the journey.

As previously stated, I remember looking at Baby Joseph everyday wishing that I could hold him, but it would be several weeks before this would happen. His little body was so frail that he couldn't be handled much, accept by the nurses and doctors. The first time we heard him sneeze was like Christmas! I remember looking at Joseph and his head nurse saying, "Oh my, was that a sneeze?" The nurse confirmed that yes, indeed, our little man had sneezed.

The day that I was able to hold him for the first time was unexplainable! I prepared to have the skin of our baby touching my skin and I declare it was breathtaking. I recall sitting in a big rocking chair (which is called a Kangaroo Chair in the NICU world) next to his incubator, while his nurse arranged all of his lines. When she placed him on my chest, I melted. He looked at me, I looked at him and it was love at first sight!

Finally, I was afforded the awesome opportunity to hold my son. As time went on, Joseph and I were able to hold baby Joseph, change his diapers and take his temperature. The March of Dimes support group volunteers were extremely helpful during this journey. Their weekly gatherings were a great encouragement to us and ignited our hope and faith that things would turn out fine. One of their volunteers even blessed us with a few photo sessions with baby Joseph, so that we could keep the memories of his stay in the hospital.

Additionally, we linked hearts with an amazing family from Whatcom County, (Jo Rust and Robin Rust Day) who were championing hope for their beloved Nathan - Joseph's roommate. We shared times of great triumph and travail. They will forever be dear to our hearts.

We would read "Psalm 91" to Baby Joseph daily and I would sing to him. A few of my favorite songs were "You're Beautiful" by James Blunt and "Amazing Grace" by John Newton.

There were many highs and lows that occurred while on this journey. There was one day that the doctor told us they saw a brain bleed, which can be common amongst preemies. After much prayer and a few tests, the report came back that the bleed was no longer present. I (Joseph) am also reminded of a weekend when Baby Joseph's primary nurse, Sabrena, called me at work and said, "Joseph is not doing well all of a sudden!" She went on to say she had run a battery of tests and done a myriad of exams and couldn't figure out why he was faltering so swiftly. I asked her honestly how Joseph was doing on a scale of 100, she gingerly responded "around 40%". I was scheduled to speak in Alaska for an International Conference, nonetheless, Baby Joseph's health and well-being was my priority. Pam and I stayed at the hospital the entire weekend. Friday was the initial call and by early Saturday morning, Joseph seemed to be coming around.

Due to the progress of our "comeback kid," Pam and I discussed that I would go to Alaska and return on a "Red Eye" flight to fulfill my commitment. The doctors gave me the "green light" and I was headed to Alaska. I literally remember leaning over to the incubator whispering, "Baby Joseph, can I go to Alaska and come back in a few hours?" Instantly, Baby Joseph's vitals tanked and the medical staff was back to revitalizing him.

About four hours later, one of the medical directors came around the corner and literally scratched his head and said, "Is this the same kid?" Now, Pam and I are fully aware it was just a personality trait that Joseph exercises when he wants his way – better known as a "temper tantrum". LOL! I think it most notable that we remained resilient in our faith during Baby Joseph's most critical few days on his journey. We've learned along the way if you keep the lens of life's circumstances positive; you will keep the fog off of the lenses from blurring your vision.

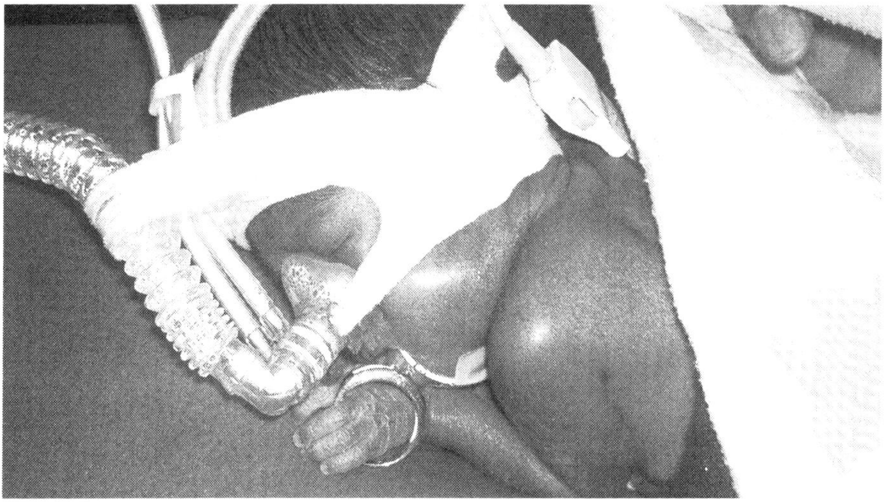

Chapter Seven

Finally Home

Upon concluding a two week tenure in the PICU (Pediatric Intensive Care Unit) to confidently bring Baby Joseph home without oxygen, we were finally released from the hospital with a 32 page discharge packet trusting him to our care for life. What an awesome moment, as we had been supported for 105 days by trained medical staff and now it was up to us to rely on the grace of God and parental instincts in raising our little champion. First venture would be traveling home twenty-two miles south, combining the responsibility of now his care and safety.

Big Joseph had to build the courage to navigate our journey home on Interstate 5 with hundreds of cars zooming by, as we took our time. A bitter sweet moment was to bring him home, while simultaneously introducing him to the fast pace of life. We finally arrived home safely, but unfortunately children don't come with instruction manuals. However, we did our best to settle as a family of three; fervently observing every move he made, as of course, anyone in our shoes would be slightly apprehensive.

We were blessed with a wonderful Village of family and friends that supported us every step of the way. There was really nothing that we needed or desired that we didn't have thanks to their love, kindness and support. Even after bringing Baby Joseph home, it was some time before he could go to public places; with the exception of doctor's appointments. We made the best out of being inside the house.

I recall going to Baby Joseph's first doctor's appointment. Once we arrived and got checked in, he began to get fussy and started crying. I asked Big Joseph to pass me the diaper bag, so that I could get his pacifier or bottle and to our surprise, there was no diaper bag! The staff laughed with us and sweetly asked, "Is this your first baby?" We humbly replied, "Yes." We were so caught up in getting all of the paperwork, getting the baby in his car seat and trying to be on time that we totally forgot to grab the diaper bag. Who does that? We did! Thank God the doctor's office was inside the hospital and the staff had the items that we needed.

Due to the circumstances that our journey presented, our God-Sister Renolda Grant notified one of our local news stations about our story. They called and gave us a heads up that they would be arriving to our home in 45 minutes to interview us. I immediately began scrambling for the most adorable outfit within reach for Baby Joseph. In a matter of hours, it was lights, camera, action! Baby Joseph was a "natural" for television. A few weeks later, we again were contacted by a local television show about appearing as a guest to share our journey.

To this day, people near and far ask if we're the couple with the "Preemie Story"; they are always amazed to see how much Baby Joseph has grown and developed. During those interviews, we made a very special announcement. Stay tuned for details in the next chapter!!!

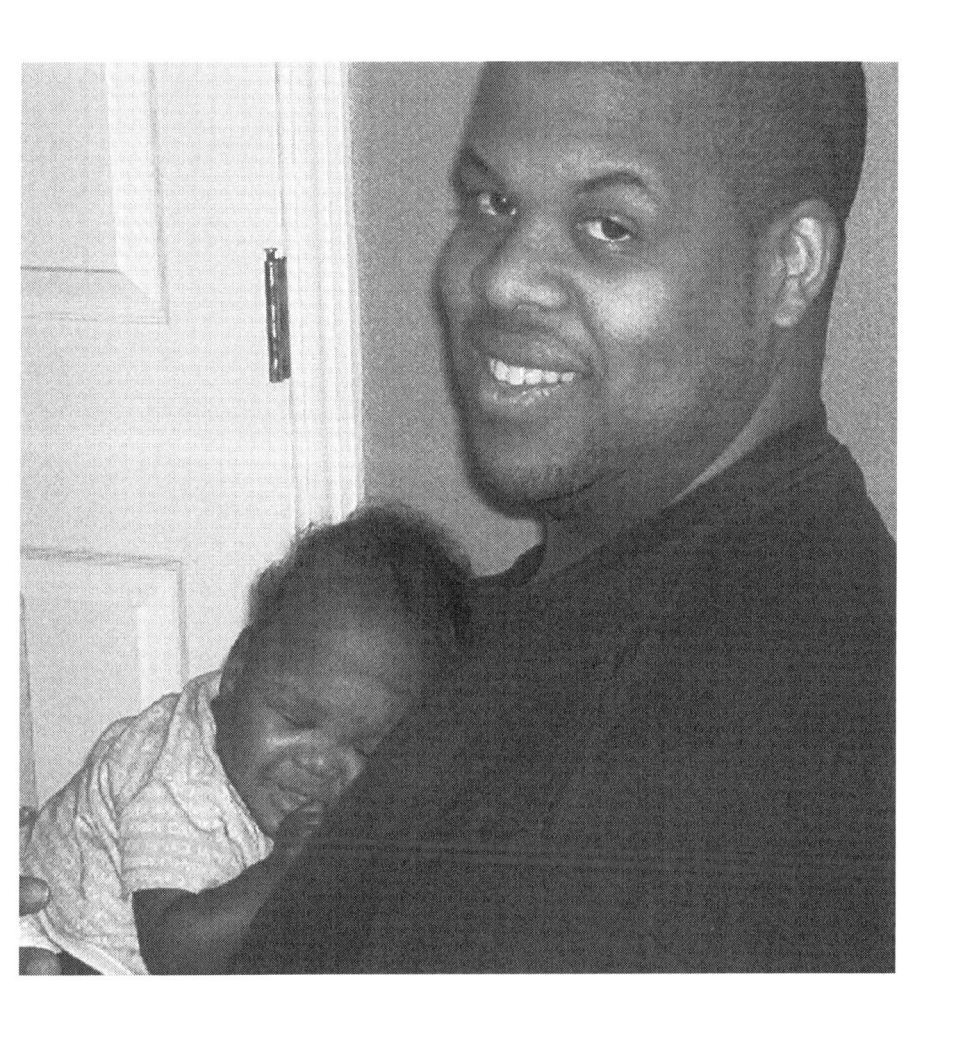

Chapter Eight

An Encore Performance

The Announcement??? Drum roll please… "We are now expecting our second child!" The same couple that was told they would never conceive is now pregnant AGAIN! We were absolutely ecstatic to learn of the news; however, one can only imagine the overwhelming potential of Baby Joseph's journey being repeated. I was referred to Perinatal medicine (a special team of doctors for high risk pregnancies). After discussing this pregnancy, it was determined that I would need a cerclage surgically placed earlier in the pregnancy term. Juggling the uncertainties of Baby Joseph's development, we were a bit perplexed as to how we would manage another pregnancy and potentially a special needs child. Baby Joseph was being tested developmentally at extensive rates! We desired to be pro-active in supporting his developmental needs. Bi-weekly, "Birth to Three" would come to our home and engage Baby Joseph through a battery of tests and activities. He was being evaluated with tasks surrounding fine motor skills and neurological development.

In July of 2009, we welcomed Josiah Alfred Bowman (who was full term) into our family. He and Baby Joseph are literally one year and three days apart. Some might call them "Irish Twins". The boys grew and developed rapidly. I (Pam) found myself being out numbered, until about fifteen months after Josiah's arrival; we welcomed Jewell Mone't Latrice Bowman (The Princess) into the family. Now Mommy had a little company. We went from ten years with no children to three children in three years! I'm not sure what you would call this, but we call it a miracle! Since the arrival of Baby Joseph, there has never been a dull moment in our home. We went from people asking us what was taking us so long to have children to now asking when we would stop!

Joseph is currently eight with the wit and personality of a congressman. Josiah is seven and a future scholar-athlete in the making, Jewell is-six and my if there is such thing as a "scholar-diva," she fits the bill. You would pay money to see the Bowman children in action! Hmmmm, let's see, "Live With The Bowman's" sounds like a really cool "Reality TV Series."

Chapter Nine

PLAYING WITH FATE: YOU WON'T BELIEVE IT!

After the birth of Jewell, we decided three was enough – despite a dream I (Joseph) had about two angels, exhausted and out of breath. Accompanying them was a young man about seventeen-years-old with beautiful hair and beautiful eyes. When the angel caught his breath, he said to me, "Meet Joshua." Another instance was a service we attended and the speaker called my wife and I forward and said we would have three sons. We were absolutely convinced that he saw three children and erred about the third son. Then, I (Pam) had dream about a little chubby boy running across the street and literally feeling the panic for his safety, as he let go of my hand solely focused on his targeted destination.

Shortly after sharing this dream with Joseph, I was invited to speak at a conference in Baltimore, MD. While on the trip, I hadn't thought about the dream at all, probably because I was focused on my assignment. After speaking that Sunday, a sweet young lady came up to me and shared some words that quickly made me think. She said, "I know this is going to sound crazy, but as you spoke and prayed for the congregants, all I could see was you pregnant." I smiled and very kindly told her that she couldn't have seen that and possibly what she saw was me pregnant with a multi-platinum Grammy award winning single! When Joseph and I were on the plane headed back home, I shared her words with him. We both looked at each other and laughed and then almost cried! I hated to admit it, but her words had pierced my heart in a very peculiar way. Even with us using protection and being cautious, deep inside the chances of this being true became very real.

Of course, children are a blessing from God and we were grateful for our three. I mean heck, according to man, we weren't scheduled to have any. Talking about beating the odds! Now my (Joseph) prayer was that our wallet would get pregnant literally–three babies in car seats and diapers! Costco welcomes us warmly every time we enter the warehouse. So of course, we began our research on the most responsive and safest birth control on the market.

I (Joseph) felt it my duty to share in the pain as my beautiful wife champion birthed three miracle children. I decided to have a vasectomy and finalize the journey of the Bowman offspring. The surgery only cost me fifteen minutes and 800 oz of pride – but I made it – fellas, you know what I mean. I followed the doctors' instructions and went to light-duty, and let me tell you, I enjoyed every minute of it. I returned six weeks later, as ordered by the doctor to test the fate of my severed VAS to find out I was more fertile after the procedure than when I came initially.

In the meantime, I was regulated to prophylactics – literally a "Trojan Man," as our efforts rendered us no gain to this point. I returned for a second surgery two months later, this time a fifteen minute procedure lasted forty-five minutes. Wait Fellas – DON'T CANCEL YOUR SCHEDULED PROCEDURE – this is just my story. 97% of vasectomy procedures last around fifteen minutes and are 99% effective (Bib). The doctor performing the surgery is a renowned university professor who has taught hundreds of doctors the art of vasectomy. He looked me in the eye and said, "Mr. Bowman, you're playing with fate – check your mailbox for a reimbursement, I can't fix you!"

I know some of you super smart people are saying why didn't I (Pam) just get a microscopy tubal ligation (tubes tied)? In all honesty, the insurance only allowed a certain number of medical occurrences per calendar year and I had reached my limit. For those of you reading who millionaires, this part of the story is not relevant to you (smile).

While determining a resolution, I (Joseph) continued sneaking around the corner at Wal-Mart to the "pleasure" aisle. Keep in mind, we live, pastor a church, and our kids attend school all in a five-mile radius, so the likelihood of simultaneously shopping with-someone we know is almost guaranteed. I cannot explain the mental pressure of arriving at the cash register being spotted and someone looking into my cart and asking the proverbial question with their eyes, "What are you doing with those in your cart?" Funny story now!

I failed to mention through all of this, Pam and I are no "spring chickens," born in the mid 70's, we were swiftly welcoming 40. I must say, we are still "pretty hot" looking, but in all reality, aging gracefully. During our time of waiting, I (Pamela) remember praying and asking God if we could make a deal. (As if He's not the master of the Universe and has time to play let's make a deal with me) but I requested that He would allow me to birth all of our children by the age of 40 and not a day, minute or second later. I was reassured that my request would be granted. I just could NOT imagine having a story anywhere near that of *the* biblical character Sarah. We SUPRISINGLY welcomed the fourth and final "Little" Bowman into the world on August 24th, 2013 – Joshua Gabriel Bowman! Just a few months before my (Pamela) 40th Birthday!

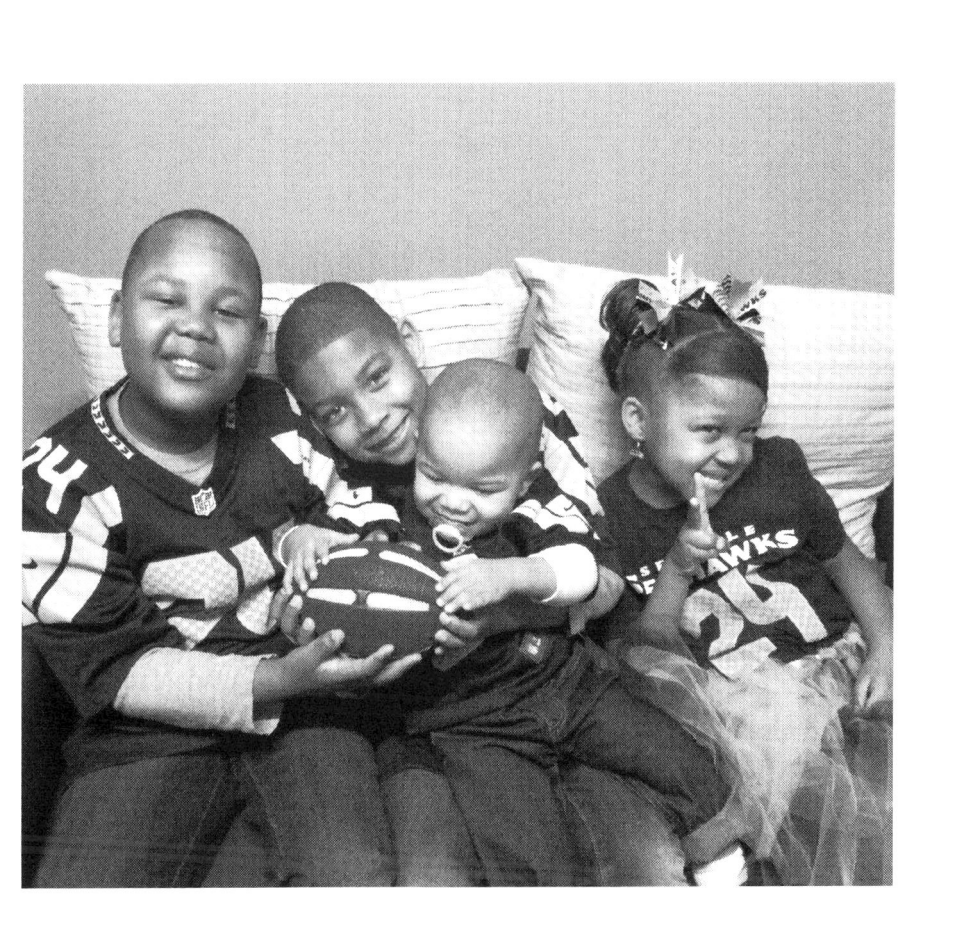

Chapter Ten

Never Give Up: Promise Keeper

Speaking from the heart of a woman; I would like to take this time to encourage every woman that has been told that it is impossible for you to conceive children. I know firsthand what it feels like to constantly hear the word "NO" regarding something that you want so badly. I also know the humiliation, guilt, sadness, pain and sometimes even the anger that can come along with it. I clearly remember dreading when Mother's Day would come around. Not because I hadn't been blessed with a wonderful Mother, Mother in love/law, Grandmother's, God Mother's and other powerful women that had made great investments into my life, but the fact still remained that I wasn't a Mother.

As a couple, we did our best to stand upright before God, while loving each other, serving God, serving people and community, and specifically, investing into the lives of young people. There were countless sleepless nights, nights where my tears became my pillow and times where the pain was so deep that I had almost become numb and upset. I had witnessed so many miracles for other people and had even experienced God answering prayers that I had prayed specifically for others and He did exactly what was requested. I almost grew weary during my process of waiting, BUT there was always-hope and faith that God would perform a miracle on our behalf!

I clearly recall Joseph and me volunteering in the homeless feeding kitchen at our former church and on that day, I felt a press to spend time in prayer. I grabbed my Bible and a hymnal and went into the main sanctuary and lay at the altar. I prayed a very personal and forthright prayer to my Heavenly Father. There were no big words, only the pureness and simplicity of my heart. I began to pray and read the Word of God highlighting His promises aloud. He said that I was more than a conquer, the head and not the tail, and that with Him, all things were possible.

After laying my heart out before Him, I began to sing hymns of encouragement. I sang songs like, "I Know It Was The Blood," "There Is Power In The Blood," "Glory To His name," "Softly and Tenderly," "Tis So Sweet To Trust In Jesus" and so many others. Because music is such a great part of me and I believe in the power of prayer, I grabbed a hold of what was most dear to me. The more I prayed and sang, the better I felt. It wasn't a temporary "good feeling," but I got up from the altar knowing without a shadow of a doubt that there was a miracle with my name written all over it. I wiped my tears, held my head up and began to thank God in advance for what He was going to do. I knew from that night on, as never before, that Joseph and I would conceive a baby. It was when I stopped worrying and wondering when and how this was going to happen that it happened!

The Promise: Prematurely Delayed

A message from the Man Cave: Fellas, we are wired warriors in the sense of making sure we FIGHT for everything, especially pertaining to our wives and kids. Have you ever had that gut-wrenching feeling of helplessness? The inability to make things better or just feeling downright cheated? I yelled to God – "Hey Man, You said, "… Be fruitful and multiply, and fill the earth, and subdue it; and rule over the fish of the sea and over the birds of the sky and over every living thing that moves on the earth." (Gen. 1:28) I felt the ethereal - larger than life – "Yeah God, You Got This! Right?"

One of the classic mysteries of God is His awesomeness, yet His ambiguous, "I am with you always!" Please don't misunderstand me; I never doubted His ability to perform a miracle; however, if He chose not to "deliver" for us, I would never defame His character as Creator of the Universe. Nonetheless, in all my believing, I was still in search for the answer when my broken wife asked me the earth shattering question, "Do You Think It Will Ever Happen For Us?" That question was soon followed by, "What's Your Perspective On All Of This?" Hey guys, I freakin' talk for a living and I had no response – nada – zilch – nothing. In that moment, all I could do was hold my loving bride close and my words became "sign language" by the affection in my arms. One day, it came to me so profoundly! "Pam sings too well to be Barren" – the gospel according to St. Joe – Chapter 44 – Verse 3. Lol! In all reality, there was a verse I referenced Isaiah:

"Shout for joy, O barren one, you who have borne no child; Break forth into joyful shouting and cry aloud, you who have not travailed; For the sons of the desolate one will be more numerous Than the sons of the married woman," says the LORD. Isaiah 54:1

I came upstairs and confidently shared unconfidently, "Your songs to the Lord – disqualifies you from Barrenness." She looked at me with such an assurance, as if it was gonna be alright. Fellas, as much as we are sought after for solutions, we must seek God for His answers pertaining to our lives. GO – FIGHT – WIN with HIM!!!

Whatever you do, DON'T GIVE UP – your dream/aspiration may be a business or a career, whatever it is. YOU CAN SUCCEED. Often, life seems to be equally "prosperous" and "painful"! I can recall each of our children being born; evolving through the contractions with Pam (sort of) and the joys we shared upon meeting the little person we so long awaited. To deepen the thought of my point - "contractions" and "delivery" were equally "pain" and "prosperity" in one moment, but what it manifested should be our focus. I am confident God is going to manifest a greater level of grace and prosperity- abundance and resources - Joy and Peace! You should EXPECT IT! We have prayed for couples all over the United States, agreed with them in faith. One couple was pregnant ten days later! It took us ten years; however, the Lord works according to His will. Who's to say you too could be a catalyst to something, or someone, greater than you?

Turn to the Next Chapter in YOUR BOOK–prepare for newness and determine you will successfully conquer all the possible challenges that present themselves as obstacles. After Baby Joseph was born at 24 weeks, Pam was ordered to have a MC. Once the cerclage was in, love making was out. The irony is love making was "in," because we shared something deeper than the act of sex. So prior to asking for a blessing, prepare yourself for all that it comes with.

The most sacred advice we can offer is to keep sacred the family bond. Without a doubt, focus on what matters most – God, Family (Spouses and Kids, in that order.) Be well assured that you are not alone. God is with you and we are with you. May you live a prosperous and healthy life!

About the Authors

Joseph & Pamela Bowman are the founding pastors of Integrity Life Church (Federal Way, WA). More importantly, the Bowman's are in love with each other and simply adore their 4 children. Affectionately known as Joe & Pam, together they aspire to develop leaders. The Bowman's are gifted communicators, contributors to several philanthropic causes and Pamela is a dynamic singer/songwriter.

Scriptures (NASB)

Psalm 91

(New American Standard)

Security of the One Who Trusts in the LORD.
1 He who dwells in the shelter of the Most High Will abide in the shadow of the Almighty.
2 I will say to the LORD, "My refuge and my fortress, My God, in whom I trust!"
3 For it is He who delivers you from the snare of the trapper And from the deadly pestilence.
4 He will cover you with His pinions, And under His wings you may seek refuge; His faithfulness is a shield and bulwark.
5 You will not be afraid of the terror by night, Or of the arrow that flies by day;
6 Of the pestilence that stalks in darkness, Or of the destruction that lays waste at noon.
7 A thousand may fall at your side And ten thousand at your right hand, But it shall not approach you.
8 You will only look on with your eyes And see the recompense of the wicked.
9 For you have made the LORD, my refuge, Even the Most High, your dwelling place.
10 No evil will befall you, Nor will any plague come near your tent.
11 For He will give His angels charge concerning you, To guard you in all your ways.
12 They will bear you up in their hands, That you do not strike your foot against a stone.
13 You will tread upon the lion and cobra,

The young lion and the serpent you will trample down.
14 "Because he has loved Me, therefore I will deliver him; I will set him securely on high, because he has known My name.
15 "He will call upon Me, and I will answer him; I will be with him in trouble; I will rescue him and honor him.
16 "With a long life I will satisfy him And let him see My salvation."

ISAIAH 54:1

(NEW AMERICAN STANDARD)

The Fertility of Zion

1 "Shout for joy, O barren one, you who have borne no child; Break forth into joyful shouting and cry aloud, you who have not travailed; For the sons of the desolate one will be more numerous Than the sons of the married woman," says the LORD.

GENESIS 1:28

(NEW AMERICAN STANDARD)

God blessed them; and God said to them, "Be fruitful and multiply, and fill the earth, and subdue it;

and rule over the fish of the sea and over the birds of the sky and over every living thing that moves on the earth."

Bibliography

Diethylstilbestrol

From about 1940 to 1970, DES was given to pregnant women in the mistaken belief it would reduce the risk of pregnancy complications and losses. In 1971, DES was shown to cause a rare vaginal tumor in girls and women who had been exposed to this drug *in utero*. The United States Food and Drug Administration subsequently withdrew DES from use in pregnant women. Follow-up studies have indicated DES also has the potential to cause a variety of significant adverse medical complications during the lifetimes of those exposed.

1. Office of Research on Women's Health, NIH, DHHS (March 2006)."Status of Research on Uterine Fibroids (leiomyomata uteri) at the National Institutes of Health". United States National Institutes of Health.

Vasectomy

Vasectomy is the most reliable practical method of permanent contraception. However, vasectomy failures have been reported. Most sources estimate the occurrence of undesired pregnancy following vasectomy to be approximately 1 in 2,000 cases.19-21 This failure rate of less than 0.1% compares favorably with the 1.85% failure rate associated with tubal ligation.22

Peterson HB, Xia Z, Hughes JM, et al. The risk of pregnancy after tubal sterilization: findings from the US Collaborative

Review of Sterilization. Am J Obstet Gynecol. 1996; 174(4):1161-1168; discussion 1168-1170.

A **McDonald Cerclage**, described in 1957 is the most common, and is essentially a purse string stitch used to cinch the cervix shut; the cervix stitching involves a band of suture at the upper part of the cervix while the lower part has already started to efface. This cerclage is usually placed between 12 weeks and 14 weeks of pregnancy. The stitch is generally removed around the 37th week of gestation.[5]

1. "Cervical Cerclage". American Pregnancy Association. Retrieved 2013-06-27.

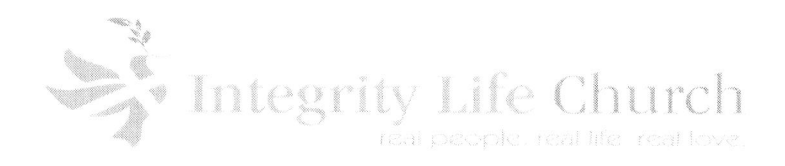

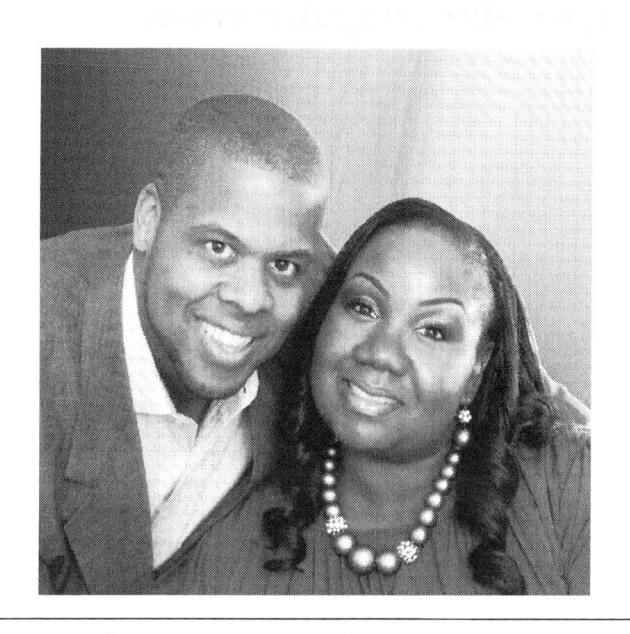

Integrity Life Church
real people. real life. real love.

INTEGRITY LIFE CHURCH
2020 S. 314TH ST
FEDERAL WAY, WA 98003

FOLLOW US ON FB AT INTEGRITY LIFE CHURCH

FOLLOW US ON TWITTER @ILC4LIFE

Made in the USA
San Bernardino, CA
28 October 2015